Basics of clinical laboratory analysis

Part 1: Liver and kidney function tests

Ayman Saber Mohamed

ISBN: 1543268870
ISBN-13: 978-1543268874

DEDICATION

I dedicate my book to my family and many friends. A special feeling of gratitude to my loving parents, Saber Mohamed, Karema Ramadan and my wife Hanan Farag whose words of encouragement and push for tenacity ring in my ears. I dedicate this work and give special thanks to my aunt Dr. Sohair R. Fahmi..

CONTENTS

ACKNOWLEDGMENTS

Firstly, I thank Allah for his grace, his success and his generosity. I take this opportunity to express my profound gratitude and deep regards to Dr. Sohair R. Fahmi, for supervising the present work, his guidance, monitoring and constant encouragement during the work. I would like to express my sincere gratitude to Dr. Amel Mahmoud Ali Soliman, for her supervision, valuable advices, stimulating suggestions through this work.
Special thanks to Prof. Dr. Mohamed Assem Said Marie, for his help and support.
I deeply thank my family for their love, support and encouragement through the work

INTRODUCTION

Clinical Laboratory Tests

Clinical laboratory tests are medical procedures to test specimens of blood, urine, or other tissues or substances from a patient.

Medical laboratory testing plays a crucial role in the detection, diagnosis and treatment of disease in patients. Laboratory tests help determine the presence, extent, or absence of disease and monitor the effectiveness of treatment.

Medical laboratory scientists analyze test results and relay them to physicians. They perform complex chemical, biological, hematological, immunologic, microscopic and bacteriological tests, requiring significant analytical and independent judgment.

Patient preparation for blood tests

- Before your test, follow all required steps for your particular laboratory test.
- The following patient instructions are intended to help you collect the correct specimen for the tests ordered by your clinicians.
- The preparation depend on type of test as the following:
1. **Lipid Profile**
   Patient should fast for 12 hours before blood collection.
   Fasting should be no food or drink except for water.

2. Blood Glucose

- Fasting blood sugar (FBS)

  For a fasting blood sugar test, do not eat or drink anything other than water for at least 8 hours before the blood sample is taken.

  If you have diabetes, your doctor may ask you to wait until you have had your blood collected before taking your morning dose of insulin or diabetes medicine.

- **2-hour Postprandial (post eat) blood sugar**: For a 2-hour postprandial test, you need to have your blood collected exactly 2 hours after a regular lunch.

- **Random blood sugar (RBS):**

  No special preparation is required before having a random blood sugar test.

3. Glucose Tolerance Test (Non-Pregnant)

- Patient should be fasting for 8 hours (no food or drink, except for water).

- A fasting blood specimen will be drawn and tested. You will then be given a glass of glucose drink. Your blood will be drawn once each hour or each half hour after you finish the drink. The number of hours may vary from 2 to 4.

4. **Prenatal Glucose Tolerance Tests**

For our pregnant patients your physician may order glucose tolerance testing during your pregnancy.

a) **50 Gram 1 Hour Glucose Tolerance Test (Gestational Diabetes Screen)**

- No special patient preparation is required.
- This test is done without regard to the time of day or time of last meal.
- You do not need to fast before this test is given.
- You will be given a glucose drink and your blood will be drawn one hour after you finish the drink.
- Please allow at least 1 ½ hours for this test to be completed.

b) **100 Gram 3 Hour Glucose Tolerance Test (Gestational Diabetes)**

- This test should be performed in the morning after an overnight fast of at least 8 hours and after at least 3 days of unrestricted diet and activity.
- A blood specimen will be drawn and tested.
- You will then be given a glucose drink.
- Your blood will be drawn once each hour after you finish the drink for three hours.
- This test will be completed in 4 hours

5. **Vitamin B12 And Folate**

   A fasting specimen (no food or drink, except for water) for 12- 14 hours before blood is drawn is preferable but not mandatory.

6. **C-Peptide**

   Patient should be fasting (no food or drink, except for water) for 12-14 hours before blood is drawn.

7. **Digoxin Level**

   Blood should be drawn 6-8 hours after the last dose of digoxin was taken. Mention the time of drug dose.

8. **Iron Study**

   No specific preparation required. Age and blood transfusion history if any, should be informed.

9. **Apolipoproteins A1/B Test**

   14 hours fasting is required, no liquids except water.

CHAPTER 1: LIVER FUNCTION TESTS

Liver function tests are blood tests used to help diagnose and monitor liver disease or damage. The tests measure the levels of certain enzymes and proteins in your blood.

Some of these tests measure how well the liver is performing its normal functions of producing protein and clearing bilirubin, a blood waste product. Other liver function tests measure enzymes that liver cells release in response to damage or disease. Abnormal liver function test results don't always indicate liver disease.

The liver function test measures the levels of different substances that are excreted by the liver such as:

Test	Sample	Normal range
Alanine Transaminase (ALT)	Serum	0–35 U/L
Aspartate Transaminase (AST)	Serum	0–35 U/L
Alkaline phosphatase (ALP)	Serum	36–92 U/L
Gamma-glutamyl transferase (GGT)	Serum	8–78 U/L
Total bilirubin	Serum	0.3–1.2 mg/dL
Direct bilirubin	Serum	0–0.3 mg/dL
Total protein	Serum	0.3–1.2
Albumin	Serum	3.5–5.5 g/dL
5'-Nucleotidase	Serum	4–11.5 U/L
Prothrombin Time (PT)	Plasma	11–13 sec
International Normalized Ratio (INR)	Plasma	2.0–3.0

1. <u>Serum transaminases enzymes</u>

Serum transaminases enzymes play a key role in animal amino acid metabolism. Serum aminotransferases activities are considered as sensitive indicators of hepatic injury. Under normal circumstances, these enzymes reside within the cells of the liver. But when the liver is injured, these enzymes are spilled into the blood stream. The elevated activities of these enzymes are indicative of cellular leakage and loss of the functional integrity of the cell membrane in the liver.

1.1. Alanine Transaminase (ALT) or Glutamate-Pyruvate Transaminase (GPT)

ALT isozymes are found in the cytosol and mitochondria of liver, kidney, skeletal and cardiac muscle. The largest pool of ALT is in the cytosol of hepatic parenchymal cells. Cytosolic ALT is associated with the utilization of pyruvate in glycolysis, while mitochondrial ALT is involved in the conversion of alanine to pyruvate for gluconeogenesis.

Glutamic acid   Pyruvic acid   Alpha-ketoglutaric acid   Alanine

ALT activity in the liver is about 3000 times that of serum activity.

6

Thus, in the case of hepatocellular injury or death, release of ALT from damaged liver cells increases measured serum ALT activity. So, serum ALT activity has been regarded as a reliable and sensitive marker of liver disease.

Clinical significance

a) **Increased activity in case of:**
- Liver diseases (acute viral hepatitis, toxic liver disease, alcohol-toxic hepatitis, sepsis, liver cirrhosis, liver metastases etc.)
- Gallbladder and biliary tract diseases (cholangitis, biliary colic)
- Myocardial diseases (heart failure with congestion of blood in the liver)
- Reye's syndrome therapeutic application of bovine or porcine heparin etc.

b) **Decreased activity in case:**
- Vitamin B6 deficiency

1.2. Aspartate Transaminase (AST) or Glutamate-Oxaloacetate Transaminase (GOT)

AST is found in both the cytosol and mitochondria of hepatocytes, but high tissue levels are also found in the heart, skeletal muscle, kidney, brain, and pancreas. Hence, when found in the blood, AST is considered a sensitive indicator of mitochondrial damage, especially in the hepatic centrilobular regions which are particularly sensitive to liver injury.

glutamate   oxaloacetate   aspartate   α-ketoglutarate

In acute hepatocellular injury, serum AST levels usually rise immediately, reaching a higher level than ALT initially, due to the high activity of AST in hepatocytes and its release with liver injury.

Clinical significance

a) Increased activity in case of:

- Liver diseases (acute viral hepatitis, toxic liver disease, alcohol-toxic hepatitis, sepsis, decompensated liver cirrhosis, liver metastases etc.)
- Gallbladder and biliary tract diseases
- Myocardial diseases (heart failure with congestion of blood in the liver)
- Reye's syndrome therapeutic application of bovine or porcine heparin etc.

b) Decreased activity in case:

- Vitamin B6 deficiency

2. Alkaline phosphatase (ALP)

The alkaline phosphatase (ALP) is from the enzymes that cause loss of the phosphorus group from many types of molecules, including nucleotides, proteins, and alkaloids, which is effective in several tissues, including bone, liver, kidney, bowel, lung, and placenta in addition to the reproductive system. ALP is an enzyme that excreted normally via bile through the liver and involves in an active transport across the capillary wall. Optimum pH: 8 – 9.

4-nitrophenylphosphate + H₂O → (ALP) → phosphate group + 4-nitrophenolate

Clinical significance

a) ALP levels may be increased in case of:

- Obstruction of the bile duct (due to gall stones, cancer, or other causes)
- Liver conditions, such as cancer, cirrhosis, or hepatitis
- Paget's disease - characterized by abnormal breakdown and regrowth of weaker bones, leading to pain and fractures

- Osteoblastic (bone-forming) bone tumors
- Metastatic bone tumors - cancers that have spread to the bone from other areas
- Hyperparathyroidism (overactive parathyroid gland)
- Rickets, due to vitamin D deficiency
- Conditions, such as ulcerative colitis (an autoimmune disease characterized by inflammation of the large bowel), lymphoma (a type of blood cancer involving lymphocytes), heart failure, and some bacterial infections

b) ALP levels may be decreased in case of:

- Hypophosphatasia: a genetic disorder with abnormal bone metabolism
- Wilson's disease : a genetic disorder characterized by copper accumulation in the body
- Zinc/protein deficiency

3. <u>Gamma-glutamyl transferase (GGT)</u>

Gamma glutamyl transferase (GGT), a microsomal enzyme that present in the membrane of the endoplasmic reticulum of the hepatocyte. GGT is contributing to the extracellular catabolism of glutathione (gamma-glutamyl-cysteinyl-glycine; GSH).

GGT catalyzes the transfer of the glutamyl group, linked

through the glutamate gamma-carboxylic acid to cysteine, to acceptor molecules including peptides, amino acids and water. As GSH is the main water-soluble antioxidant within the cell, GGT has been traditionally regarded as a component of the cell protection system against oxidative stress.

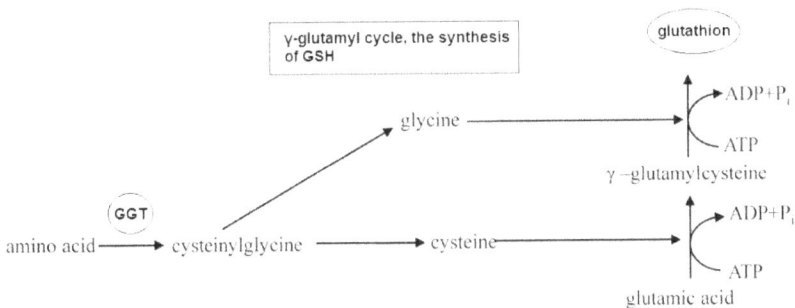

GGT expression varies considerably among normal tissues. In particular, high GGT activities are present on the luminal surface of secretory and absorptive cells, including those of bile ducts, bile canaliculi and proximal tubules of the kidney, and in endothelial cells of nervous system capillaries. GGT is carried primarily with lipoproteins and albumin. GGT is more sensitive than alkaline phosphatase (ALP) in detecting all forms of liver disease.

Clinical Significance

Elevated levels of GGT are found in conditions, such as:

- Bile duct obstruction
- Hepatitis

- Liver diseases, such as cirrhosis, or tumors, or liver damage from drug toxicity
- Alcohol abuse
- Diabetes
- Pancreatitis
- Heart failure

4. Bilirubin

Bilirubin derives from haem present in haemoglobin and is released during the breakdown of senescent erythrocytes. It is formed in the monocytic macrophages of the spleen and bone marrow and in hepatic Kupffer cells. Haem catabolism produces equimolar amounts of biliverdin, carbon monoxide, and free divalent iron. Biliverdin is subsequently reduced to bilirubin. In the blood stream bilirubin appears as a weak dianion that is almost insoluble in aqueous solutions at the physiological pH, and to a large extent bound to albumin in the circulation. Reaching the parenchymal cells of the liver, bilirubin, but not albumin, crosses the cell membrane of the hepatocyte. In the hepatocyte unconjugated bilirubin is converted to the water-soluble conjugated bilirubin and excreted into the bile.

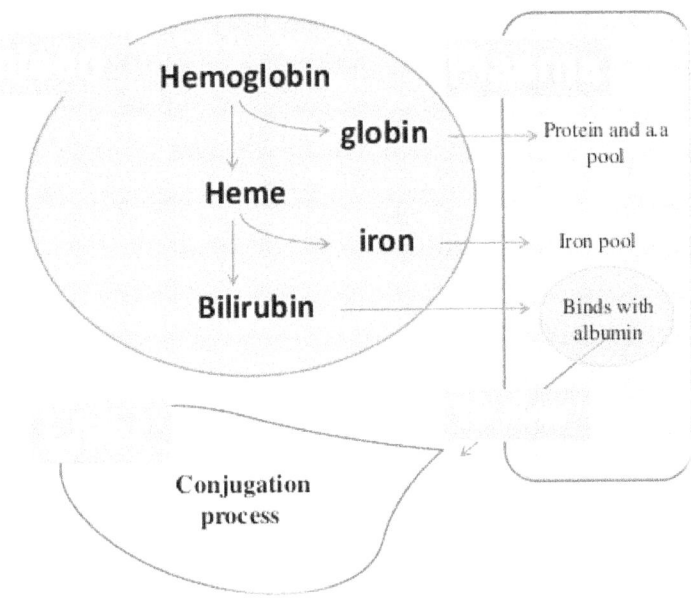

Serum bilirubin is one of the most sensitive tests employed in the diagnosis of hepatic diseases and any abnormal increase in the level of bilirubin in the serum indicates hepatobiliary disease and severe disturbance of hepatocellular.

Unconjugated bilirubin (Indirect bilirubin)	Conjugated bilirubin (Direct bilirubin)
Tightly bind to albumin	Weak bind to albumin
Water insoluble	Water soluble
Toxic	Non toxic
Cannot be excreted in urine	excreted in urine
90% of total bilirubin	10% of total bilirubin

Bilirubin is conjugated with glucuronic acid by the enzyme glucuronyltransferase, making it soluble in water:

The measurement of direct bilirubin depends on its reaction with diazosulfanilic acid to create azobilirubin. However, unconjugated bilirubin also reacts slowly with diazosulfanilic acid, so that the measured indirect bilirubin is an underestimate of the true unconjugated concentration.

Clinical Significance

a) In newborns

Bilirubin levels are higher for the first few days of life. Jaundice happens when bilirubin builds up faster than a newborn's liver can break it down and pass it from the body. Here are some reasons why:

- Newborns make more bilirubin than adults do since they have more turnovers of red blood cells.
- A newborn baby's still-developing liver might not be able to remove enough bilirubin from the blood.

b) Jaundice can also occur when more red blood cells than normal are broken down. This can be caused by:

- Erythroblastosis fetalis
- Hemolytic anemia
- Transfusion reaction

c) The following liver problems may also cause jaundice or high bilirubin levels:

- Cirrhosis
- Hepatitis
- Liver disease
- Gilbert's disease

d) The following problems with gallbladder or bile ducts may cause higher bilirubin levels:

- Biliary stricture
- Cancer of the pancreas or gallbladder
- Gallstones

5. <u>Total protein</u>

The Liver is the major source of the most the serum proteins. The liver normally comprises approximately 15% of the total protein synthesizing capacity of the body, while the remaining 85% is distributed among the other tissues. In cases where tissue protein synthesis is reduced, the liver protein-synthesizing capacity may rise up to over 30% for compensation. Conversely, once the protein synthetic capacity of the liver is affected, serum albumin levels are reduced, and, this is compensated for by proteins synthesized in extra-hepatic tissues. Thus, a balance is created, widely known as an altered albumin/globulin ratio (A/G) ratio.

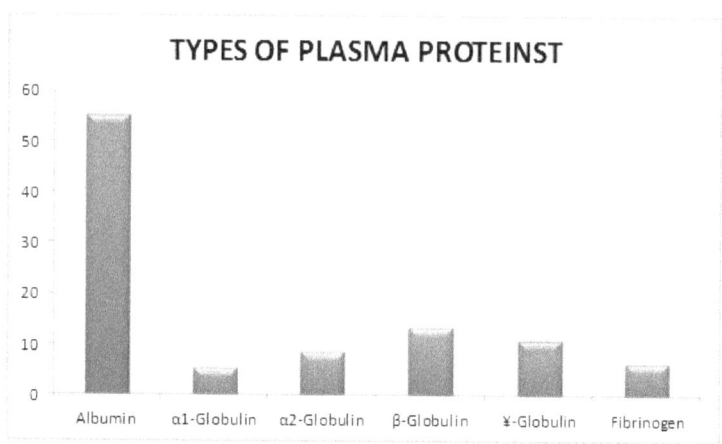

Clinical Significance

a) A low level of total protein indicates:
- Serious case of malnutrition (maybe due to a lack of insufficient absorption of proteins)
- Conditions producing malabsorption of proteins, like Celiac disease, inflammatory bowel disease, etc.
- Kidney or liver related disease.

b) A high level of total protein indicates:
- Kidney or liver related diseases
- Chronic inflammations and/or infections (viral hepatitis, HIV)
- Bone marrow disorders (multiple myeloma, etc.)

6. __Albumin__

Albumin is the most abundant circulating protein in the plasma and the most important protein synthesized by the liver. It has several important physiological and pharmacological functions as it transports metals, fatty acids, cholesterol, bile pigments, and drugs and it is a key element in the regulation of osmotic pressure and distribution of fluid between different compartments. The synthesis of albumin reflects the extent of functioning of liver cell mass. In addition, globulins constitute immunoglobulin's produced by B lymphocytes as well as α and β globulins synthesized mainly by hepatocytes. The characteristic alterations in the serum proteins in chronic liver disease, namely, hypoalbuminemia and hyperglobulinemia chiefly of the gamma fraction, have been reported by numerous studies.

Furthermore, the albumin/globulin (A/G) ratio is a biochemical parameter utilized in the interpretation of changes in serum proteins that accompany the disease. The main clinical use of the A/G ratio is when it is reduced as a result of decrease in serum albumin and the sequential increase in serum globulins. This is the classical change expected to accompany liver disease when serum albumin is decreased below normal levels.

Clinical Significance

a) Low albumin levels may indicate:

- Liver disease
- Nephrotic syndrome or nephritic syndrome, in which the kidneys are unable to prevent albumin in blood, from leaking into the urine
- Malnutrition, infection, prolonged diarrhea, and chronic illness
- In conditions where the body does not absorb and digest protein, such as Crohn's disease, Whipple's disease, or sprue
- Extensive burns
- Major surgeries
- A variety of cancers
- Decreased thyroid hormones levels
- Redistribution or changes in fluid volume of blood, due to heart failure, pregnancy, shock
- Diabetes

b) High albumin levels may indicate:

- It is commonly observed with dehydration

7. <u>5'-Nucleotidase</u>

- 5'-Nucleotidase (5'-NT) is an enzyme found in the liver. It is attached to the membranes of the liver cells
- The function of 5'-NT is to create the molecule adenosine. Adenosine is important for numerous biological functions, including energy production and signaling
- 5'-NT creates adenosine from adenosine monophosphate (AMP).

$$AMP \xrightarrow{5'\ Nucleotidase} Adenosine + P_i.$$

<u>Clinical Significance</u>

An elevated 5'-Nucleotidase may indicate:

- Cholestatic liver disease
- Secondary tumors and lymphoma of the liver
- Early biliary cirrhosis
- Inflammatory arthritis

8. **Prothrombin Time and International Normalized Ratio PT/INR Test**

- Prothrombin is the inactive form (proenzyme) of thrombin, an enzyme that forms blood clots. Thrombin helps in blood clot formation, by converting a soluble protein (fibrinogen) to its insoluble form (fibrin). The fibrins then coalesce into a blood clot

- The Prothrombin Time (PT) is a the time taken for a clot to form (or the clotting time) in a serum sample, after the necessary factors are added
- From the clotting time, an International Normalized Ratio (INR) is calculated. INR takes into account the different methods used by laboratories to measure clotting time.
- PT/INR Tests are useful for monitoring the balance between excessive and insufficient coagulability (ability to change into clots) of blood. This is essential during therapy using anticoagulants, such as metformin or heparin

Clinical Significance

a) Prolonged prothrombin time may indicate:
- Liver disorder
- Bone marrow disorder
- Vitamin K deficiency
- The individual is on anticoagulant therapy

- Collagen disorder
- Disseminated intravascular coagulation (DIC)
- Cancer
- Chronic pancreatitis
- Toxic shock syndrome
- Genetic disorders involving the clotting factors of the extrinsic and common pathways
- Lupus anticoagulants

a) Accelerated prothrombin time may indicate:

- Predisposition to clot formation within the blood vessels (thrombosis)
- Blockage of blood flow (embolism)
- Tissue damage, due to lack of blood flow (infarction)
- Multiple myeloma

CHAPTER 2: LIPID PROFILE

Lipids are a group of fats and fat-like substances that are important constituents of cells and sources of energy. Cholesterol and triglycerides are important constituents of the lipid fraction of the human body.

Cholesterol and triglycerides, being nonpolar lipid substances (insoluble in water), need to be transported in the plasma associated with various lipoprotein particles. Plasma lipoproteins are separated by hydrated density; electrophretic mobility; size; and their relative content of cholesterol, triglycerides, and protein into five major classes: chylomicrons, very-low-density lipoproteins (VLDL), intermediate-density lipoproteins (IDL), low-density lipoproteins (LDL), and high-density lipoproteins (HDL). Each particle contains a mixture of cholesterol, triglyceride, and protein, but in varying amounts unique to each type of particle. LDL contains the highest amount of cholesterol. HDL contains the highest amount of protein, VLDL and chylomicrons contain the highest amount of triglyceride.

Test	Sample	Normal range
Cholesterol	Plasma	150–199 mg/dL
Triglycerides	Serum	< 250 mg/dL
High-density lipoproteins (HDL)	Plasma	≥ 40 mg/dL
Low-density lipoproteins (LDL)	Plasma	≤ 130 mg/dL
Very low-density lipoproteins (VLDL)	Plasma	≤ 30 mg/dL

1. <u>Cholesterol</u>

Cholesterol is a kind of fatty substance that plays an important role in the human body. The body is capable of producing cholesterol and some of it is obtained from the diet.

Cholesterol helps in:

- Forming the covering of all cells (plasma membrane) in the body
- The formation of some hormones
- The production of bile acids that help in absorbing fats and some vitamins from food.

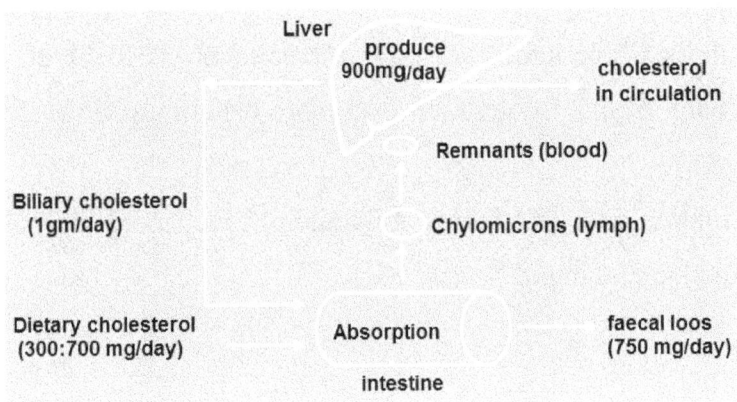

<u>Clinical significant</u>

Cholesterol Test results can be divided into 3 groups depending on the risk for heart disease:

a) **Desirable: Low risk for heart disease**

- Adults: Cholesterol level below 200 mg/dL
- Young adults: Cholesterol level below 190 mg/dL
- Children and adolescents: Cholesterol level below 170 mg/dL

b) Borderline: Moderate risk for heart disease

- Adults: Cholesterol level of 200 to 239 mg/dL
- Young adults: Cholesterol level of 190-224 mg/dL
- Children and adolescents: Cholesterol level of 170-199 mg/dL

c) High risk for heart disease

- Adults: Cholesterol level more than or equal to 240 mg/dL
- Young adults: Cholesterol level more than or equal to 225 mg/dL
- Children and adolescents: Cholesterol level more than or equal to 200 mg/dL

2. <u>High-density lipoproteins (HDL)</u>

High-density lipoprotein HDL cholesterol particle is dense compared to other types of cholesterol particles, so it's called high-density. HDL is known as the "good" cholesterol because it helps remove other forms of cholesterol from your bloodstream. Higher levels of HDL cholesterol are associated with a lower risk of heart disease because:

- HDL cholesterol scavenges and removes LDL- or "bad" cholesterol.

- HDL reduces and recycles LDL cholesterol by transporting it to the liver where it can be reprocessed.

- HDL cholesterol acts as a maintenance crew for the inner walls (endothelium) of blood vessels. Damage to the inner walls is the first step in the process of atherosclerosis, which causes heart attacks and strokes. HDL scrubs the wall clean and keeps it healthy

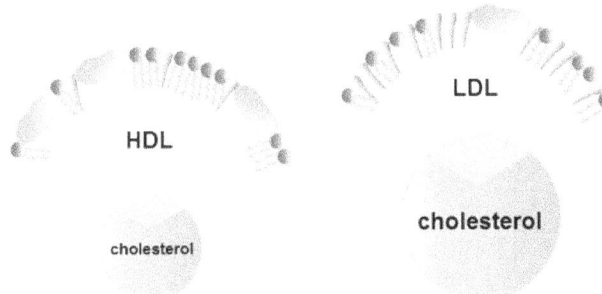

Clinical significant

a) High HDL cholesterol levels may indicate:

- Familial hyper-a-lipoprotcincmia
- Biliary cirrhosis
- Chronic hepatitis
- Tangier disease

- Chronic renal failure
- Cholestasis
- Hepatocellular disorders
- Nephrotic syndrome
- Premature coronary artery disease (CAD)

b) Low HDL cholesterol levels may indicate:

- A-ß-lipoproteinemia
- Fish eye disease
- Hypertriglyceridemia
- Chronic anemia
- Chronic pulmonary disease
- Severe hepatocellular destruction or disease
- Hyperthyroidism
- Inflammatory joint disease
- Myeloma
- Reye's syndrome

3. **Low-density lipoprotein (LDL)**

Low-density lipoprotein (LDL) carries mostly cholesterol, some protein, and minimal triglycerides throughout your circulation. These molecules are larger, less dense, and less stable than high-density lipoprotein (HDL). They readily oxidize and deposit plaques on arterial walls which are likely to clog arteries and lead to cardiovascular disease. That's why LDL is known as the "bad" cholesterol.

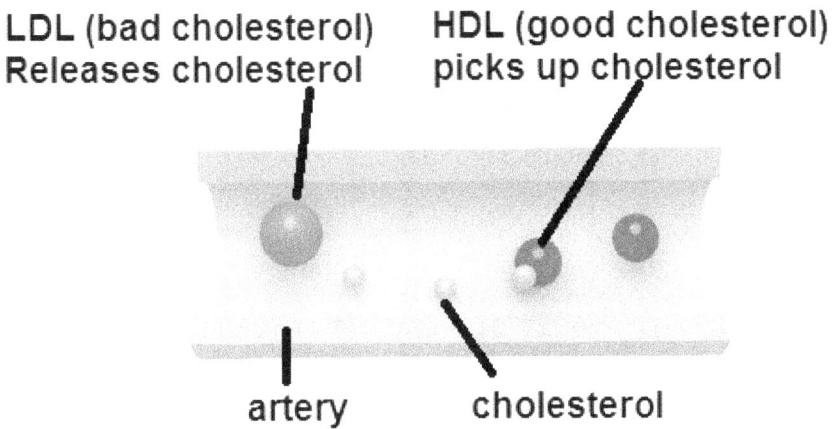

LDL (bad cholesterol) Releases cholesterol

HDL (good cholesterol) picks up cholesterol

artery   cholesterol

Clinical significant

- 25 - 100 mg/dl indicates an optimal LDL cholesterol level
- 100 - 129 mg/dl indicates a near optimal LDL level, which corresponds to a higher rate of developing symptomatic cardiovascular diseases
- 130 - 159 mg/dl indicates a borderline high LDL level, which corresponds to a high rate of developing symptomatic cardiovascular diseases
- 160 - 199 mg/dl corresponds to a high LDL level resulting in a much higher rate of developing symptomatic cardiovascular diseases
- > 200 mg/dl indicates a very high LDL level, which corresponds to highly increased rates of symptomatic cardiovascular diseases

4. <u>Very low density lipoprotein</u>

VLDL is one of the three main types of lipoproteins. VLDL contains the highest amount of triglycerides. VLDL is a type of "bad cholesterol" because it helps cholesterol build up on the walls of arteries.

<u>Clinical significant</u>

a) Increased serum LDL and VLDL cholesterol levels:

- Genetic Lipid disorders

- Bile duct blockage

- Nephrotic syndrome

- Obstructive jaundice

- Hypothyroidism

- Fat rich diet

b) Decreased serum LDL and VLDL cholesterol levels:

- Malnutrition

- Cellular necrosis of the liver

- Hyperthyroidism.

To estimate VLDL, divide the triglyceride value by 5 if the value is in mg/dL or divide by 2.2 if the value is in mmol/L

OR:

VLDL = (Total Cholesterol) – (HDL) – (LDL)

5. Triglycerides

Triglycerides are fat or lipid molecules used by the body mainly for energy storage. 95% of the adipose tissues are composed of triglycerides. The structure of triglycerides, or triacylglycerol, is that of a glycerol backbone connected to 3 fatty acid tails. There are many kinds of triglycerides, depending on the length of the fatty acids attached to glycerol. Triglycerides either meet immediate energy needs in muscles or stored as fat for future energy requirements.

Triglyceride molecule

right top: palmitic acid

right middle: oleic acid

right bottom: alpha-linolenic acid

left part = glyceryol

Point of comparison	Cholesterol	Triglycerides
Source	Dietary source. Endogenous source (liver).	Dietary source. Endogenous source (liver).
Function	Biosynthesis the cell and some hormones	Create energy

Clinical significant

a) High triglyceride levels may indicate:

- Excessive intake of dietary fats
- Sedentary lifestyle
- Diabetes
- Hypothyroidism
- Alcohol use
- Liver disease
- Pancreatic disease

b) Low triglyceride levels may indicate:

- Congenital alpha-beta-lipoproteinemia
- Malnutrition
- Hyperthyroidism

CHAPTER 3: KIDNEY FUNCTION TESTS

The routine blood and urine tests listed below may provide the first indication of a kidney problem or may be ordered if chronic kidney disease is suspected due to a person's signs and symptoms. These tests reflect how well the kidneys are removing excess fluids and wastes and some are included in the basic and comprehensive metabolic panels.

Creatinine	Sample	0.7–1.3 mg/dL
Urea	Serum	15 to 45 mg/dL
Urea nitrogen	-	8–20 mg/dL
Uric acid	Serum	2.5–8 mg/dL

1. <u>Creatinine</u>

- Creatinine is a chemical waste molecule that is generated from muscle metabolism.
- Creatinine is produced from creatine, a molecule of major importance for energy production in muscles.
- Approximately 2% of the body's creatine is converted to creatinine every day.
- Creatinine is transported through the bloodstream to the kidneys.
- The kidneys filter out most of the creatinine and dispose of it in the urine.

- Because the muscle mass in the body is relatively constant from day to day, the creatinine production rate is relatively constant.

Clinical significant

a) Increased blood creatinine levels may indicate:

- Acromegaly
- Congestive heart failure

- Dehydration
- Gigantism
- Hyperthyroidism
- Poliomyelitis
- Kidney disease, including acute and chronic kidney failure
- Rhabdomyolysis
- Shock
- Diabetes mellitus
- Nephritis
- Gout
- Multiple myeloma
- Rheumatoid arthritis
- Subacute bacterial endocarditis
- Systemic lupus erythematosus (SLE)
- Uremia
- Urinary obstruction

b) Decreased blood creatinine levels may indicate:

- Inadequate protein intake
- Severe liver disease
- Muscular dystrophy

2. Creatinine clearance

This test measures creatinine levels in both a sample of blood and a sample of urine from a 24-hour urine collection. The results are used to calculate the amount of creatinine that has been cleared from the blood and passed into the urine. This calculation allows for a general evaluation of the amount of blood that is being filtered by the kidneys in a 24-hour time period.

3. Urea

The urea is the major nitrogenous end product of protein and amino acid catabolism, produced by the liver and distributed throughout intracellular and extracellular fluid. Urea formation is influenced by a number of factors such as liver function, protein intake and rate of protein catabolism. Urea excretion also depends upon hydration status and the extent of water re-absorption as well as upon glomerular filtration rate. The most frequently determined clinical indices for estimating renal function depends upon concentration of urea in the serum.

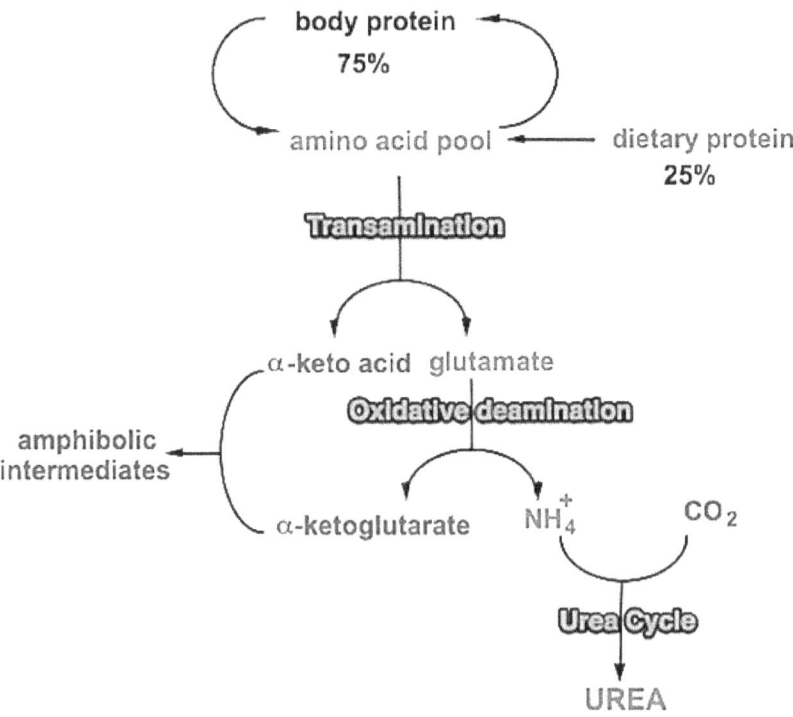

Clinical significant

a) Urea nitrogen levels are higher than normal in the following cases:

- Probable kidney malfunction or kidney failure
- Indication of high protein intake or inadequate fluid intake
- Poor blood circulation leading to less filtering of urea into urine (may be due to congestive heart failure, shock)
- Dehydration, burns, or fever
- Gastrointestinal bleeding
- Urinary tract obstruction

• Heart attack

b) Urea nitrogen levels are lower than normal in the following cases:

• Malnutrition
• Liver disease or liver damage; additional tests would be required, prior to confirming such a diagnosis
• Low protein diet
• Over-hydration

4. Uric acid

• Uric acid is a breakdown product of an important class of nitrogen-containing compounds, called purines.
• Purines make up 2 of the 4 building blocks of DNA and RNA. They also comprise other important molecules, such as ATP - the body's energy currency, cAMP - an important signaling molecule, and coenzyme A, which is essential to many chemical reactions

Uric acid

- Most purines in the body originate from cells that have died and released their DNA and RNA. A dietary intake of purine also contributes to the body's purine supply, though to a lesser extent. Common sources of purines include organ meats, beans, and yeasts (such as those present in beer)

- Increased levels of purines lead to increased uric acid levels, unless there is an abnormality associated with the body's purine degradation system. Uric acid is excreted through urine and feces. However, it may accumulate in blood, due to overproduction or impaired excretion

- Uric acid that has accumulated may deposit in the joints, causing inflammation. This is known as gout.

- Uric acid may also combine with other compounds, such as calcium, and form "stones" in the kidneys, ureters, or bladder

Clinical significant

a) Increased uric acid levels may indicate:

- Gout
- Kidney, ureter, or bladder stones
- Sudden tissue destruction as a result of starvation, or excessive exercise
- Cancer
- Chronic renal disease
- Acidosis
- Toxemia of pregnancy
- Alcoholism
- Down syndrome
- Chronic lead toxicity
- Eclampsia
- Hypertension
- Parathyroid dysfunction
- Lesch-Nyhan syndrome
- Multiple myeloma
- Anemia
- Type III hyperlipidemia

b) Decreased uric acid levels may indicate:

- Fanconi's syndrome
- Severe liver disease
- Wilson's disease

REFERENCES

1. Akanji, M. A.; Olagoke, O.A. and Oloyede, O.B. (1993): Effect of chronic consumption of metabisulphite on the integrity of the rat kidney cellular system. Toxicology, 81(3): 173–179.

2. Akanji, M. A.; Olagoke, O.A. and Oloyede, O.B. (1993): Effect of chronic consumption of metabisulphite on the integrity of the rat kidney cellular system. Toxicology, 81(3): 173–179.

3. Alibawi, F. A. N. A.; Al-Morshidy, S. Y. and Alhuweizi, A. G. (2012): The alkaline phosphatase levels in the seminal plasma and sperms of sub-fertile patients and normospermic men. Int. Con. Applied Life Sci., (ICALS2012), Turkey, September 10-12, 2012. Pp: 217-222.

4. Alibawi, F. A. N. A.; Al-Morshidy, S. Y. and Alhuweizi, A. G. (2012): The alkaline phosphatase levels in the seminal plasma and sperms of sub-fertile patients and normospermic men. Int. Con. Applied Life Sci., (ICALS2012), Turkey, September 10-12, 2012. Pp: 217-222.

5. Al-Joudi, F. S. and Wahab, N. A. (2004): The utilization of an index for serum globulin compensation in diseases associated with decreased serum albumin. Med. J. Malaysia, 59 (4): 495-501.

6. Amacher D. E. (1998): Serum transaminase elevations as indicators of hepatic injury following the administration of drugs. Regulatory Toxicol. Pharmacol. J., 27: 119- 130.

7. Bansal, V. and Schuchert, V.D. (2006): Jaundice in the Intensive Care Unit. Surg. Clin. N. Am., 86: 1495–1502.

8. Bays, H. (2002): Ezetimibe. Expert. Opin. Investig. Drugs, 11(11):1587-604.

9. Brodersen, R. (1979): Bilirubin-solubility and interaction with albumin and phospholipid. J. Biol. Chem., 254: 2364– 2369.

10. Bruille, D.; Rose, F.; Arna, M.; Melin, C. and Obled, C. (1994): Sepsis modifies the contribution of different organs to whole body protein synthesis in rats. Clin. Sci., 86 (6): 663-669.

11. Corti, A.; Franzini, M.; Paolicchi, A. and Pompella, A. (2010): Gamma-glutamyltransferase of cancer cells at the crossroads of tumor progression, drug resistance and drug targeting. Anticancer Res., 30(4):1169-1181.

12. Corti, A.; Franzini, M.; Paolicchi, A. and Pompella, A. (2010): Gamma-glutamyltransferase of cancer cells at the crossroads of tumor progression, drug resistance and drug targeting. Anticancer Res., 30(4):1169-1181.

13. Dufour, D. R.; Lott, J. A.; Nolte, F. S.; Gretch, D. R.; Koff, R. S. and Seeff, L. B. (2000): Diagnosis and monitoring of hepatic injury. Recommendations for use of

laboratory tests in screening, diagnosis and monitoring. Clin. Chem., 46 (12): 2050-2068.

14.   Edet, E. E.; Atangwho, I.J.; Akpanabiatu, M.I.; Edet, T. E.; Uboh, F.E. and Amacher-Oku. E. (2011): Effect of *Gongronema latifolium* leaf extract on some liver enzymes and protein levels in diabetic and non-diabetic rats. J. Pharm. Biomed. Sci., 1(5): 104-107.

15.   Edet, E. E.; Atangwho, I.J.; Akpanabiatu, M.I.; Edet, T. E.; Uboh, F.E. and Amacher-Oku. E. (2011): Effect of *Gongronema latifolium* leaf extract on some liver enzymes and protein levels in diabetic and non-diabetic rats. J. Pharm. Biomed. Sci., 1(5): 104-107.

16.   Emdin, M.; Pompella, A. and Paolicchi, A. (2005): Gamma-glutamyltransferase, atherosclerosis, and cardiovascular disease: triggering oxidative stress within the plaque. Circulation, 112(14): 2078 -2080.

17.   Emdin, M.; Pompella, A. and Paolicchi, A. (2005): Gamma-glutamyltransferase, atherosclerosis, and cardiovascular disease: triggering oxidative stress within the plaque. Circulation, 112(14): 2078 -2080.

18.   Froh, M.; Conzelmann, L.; Walbrun, P.; Netter, S.; Wiest, R.; Wheeler, M.D.; Lehnert, M.; Uesugi, T.; Scholmerich, Ju. and Thurman, R.G. (2007): Heme oxygenase-1 overexpression increases liver injury after bile duct ligation in rats. World J. Gastroenterol., 13 (25): 3478-3486.

19. Gowda, S.; Desai, P. B.; Kulkarni, S. S.; Hull, V. V.; Math, K. A. and Vernekar, S. N. (2010): Markers of renal function tests. N. Am. J. Med. Sci., 2 (4): 170-173.

20. Gowda, S.; Desai, P. B.; Kulkarni, S. S.; Hull, V. V.; Math, K. A. and Vernekar, S. N. (2010): Markers of renal function tests. N. Am. J. Med. Sci., 2 (4): 170-173.

21. Griffin, K. A.; Kramer, H. and Bidani, A. K. (2008): Adverse renal consequences of obesity. Am. J. Physiol. Renal Physiol., 294: 685-696.

22. Hall, P. and Cash, J. (2012): What is the Real Function of the Liver 'Function' Tests? *Ulster. Med. J.*, 81(1): 30-36

23. Hanigan, M. H. and Frierson, H. F. (1996): Immunohistochemical detection of gamma-glutamyl transpeptidase in normal human tissue. J. Histochem. Cytochem., 44: 1101-1108.

24. Hanigan, M. H. and Frierson, H. F. (1996): Immunohistochemical detection of gamma-glutamyl transpeptidase in normal human tissue. J. Histochem. Cytochem., 44: 1101-1108.

25. Hass, P. (1999): Differentiation and diagnosis of jaundice. A.A.C.N. Clinical Issues: Advanced Practice in Acute Critical Care., 10(4) :433–441.

26. Henry, J.B. and Saunders, W.B. (1996): Clinical Diagnosis and Management by Laboratory Methods, 19th Edition.

27. Herlong, H. F. (1994): Approach to the patient with abnormal liver enzymes. Hosp. Pract., 29: 32–38.

28. Kee, J. L. (2010). Laboratory and diagnostic tests with nursing implications (8th ed.). Upper Saddle River, NJ: Pearson.

29. Khalaf, A. A. A.; Mekawy, E. M.; Moawad, S. M. and Ahmed, A. M. (2009): Comparative study on the protective effect of some antioxidants against CCl_4 hepatotoxicity in rats. Egypt. J. Nat. Toxins, 6 (1): 59-82.

30. Khalaf, A. A. A.; Mekawy, E. M.; Moawad, S. M. and Ahmed, A. M. (2009): Comparative study on the protective effect of some antioxidants against CCl_4 hepatotoxicity in rats. Egypt. J. Nat. Toxins, 6 (1): 59-82.

31. Kim, W. R.; Flamm, S. L.; Di Bisceglie, A. M. and Bodenheimer, H. C. (2008): Serum activity of alanine aminotransferase (ALT) as an indicator of health and disease. Hepatology, 47(4): 1363–1370.

32. Kumar, V., Abbas, A. K., Aster, J. C., & Robbins, S. L. (2013). *Robbins basic pathology* (9th ed.). Philadelphia, PA: Elsevier/Saunders.

33. *Lab Tests Online* (2014, January 25). Retrieved March 1, 2014   from http://labtestsonline.org/understanding/analytes/pt/

34. Lightner, D.A., Reisinger, M., and Landen, G. L. (1986): On the structure of albumin- bound bilirubin-selective binding of intramolecularly hydrogen-bonded

conformational enantiomers. J. Biol. Chem., 261:6034-6038.

35. Maisels, M. J. (1999): Jaundice. In Neonatology, Pathophysiology & Management of the Newborn, eds. Avery GB, Fletcher MA, & MacDonald MG, 765-820. Lippincott Williams & Wilkins, Philadelphia

36. Martin, P. and Fridman, L.S. (1992): Assessment of liver function and diagnostic studies. In: Friedman; L.S.; Keefe; E.B. (Eds.); Hand Book of Liver disease. Churchill Livingstone; Philadelphia, 1–14.

37. Martini, F., Nath, J. L., & Bartholomew, E. F. (2012). Fundamentals of anatomy & physiology (9th ed.). San Francisco: Benjamin Cummings.

38. Martini, F., Nath, J. L., & Bartholomew, E. F. (2012). *Fundamentals of anatomy & physiology* (9th ed.). San Francisco: Benjamin Cummings.

39. Misumi, Y. (1990). Primary structure of human placental 5′-nucleotidase and identification of the glycolipid anchor in the mature form. European Journal of Biochemistry, 191(3), 563-69.

40. Muriel, P. and Escobar, Y. (2003): Kupffer cells are responsible for liver cirrhosis induced by carbon tetrachloride. J. App. Toxicol., 23(2):103-108.

41. Muriel, P. and Escobar, Y. (2003): Kupffer cells are responsible for liver cirrhosis induced by carbon tetrachloride. J. App. Toxicol., 23(2):103-108.

42. Naik, S. R. and Panda, V. S. (2008): Hepatoprotective effect of *Ginkgoselect phytosome* in rifampicin induced liver injury in rats: evidence of antioxidant activity. Fitoterapia, 79: 439-445.

43. Neuschwander-Tetri, B. A. and Caldwell, S. H. (2003): Nonalcoholic steatohepatitis: summary of an AASLD Single Topic Conference. Hepatology, 37(5): 1202-1219.

44. Rajesh, M. G. and Latha, M. S. (2004): Preliminary evaluations of the antihepatotoxic effect of Kamilari, a polyherbal formulation. J. Ethnopharmacol., 91: 99-104.

45. Rej, R. (1989): Aminotransferases in disease. Clin. Lab. Med., 9(4): 667–687.

46. Roche, M.; Rondeau, P.; Singh, N. R.; Tarnus, E. and Bourdon, E. (2008): The antioxidant properties of serum albumin. FEBS Letters, 582(13): 1783–1787.

47. Roche, M.; Rondeau, P.; Singh, N. R.; Tarnus, E. and Bourdon, E. (2008): The antioxidant properties of serum albumin. FEBS Letters, 582(13): 1783–1787.

48. Rodriguez, G.; Gallego, S.; Breidenassel, C.; Moreno, L. A. and Gottrand, F. (2010); Is liver transaminases assessment an appropriate tool for the screening of non-alcoholic fatty liver disease in at risk obese children and adolescents. Nutr. Hosp., 25(5):712-717.

49. Sakagishi, Y. (1995): Alanine aminotransferase (ALT). Japanese J. Clin. Med., 53: 1146–1150.

50. Schachter, D. (1957): Nature of the glucuronide in direct-reacting bilirubin. Sci., 126: 507–508.

51. Schafer AI. Approach to the patient with bleeding and thrombosis. In: Goldman L, Schafer AI, eds. *Cecil Medicine*. 24th ed. Philadelphia, Pa: Saunders Elsevier; 2011:chap 174

52. Schmidt, E. and Schmidt, F. W. (1990): Progress in the enzyme diagnosis of liver disease: Reality or illusion. Clin. Biochem., 23; 375– 382.

53. Sharma, A.; Hirulkar, N. B.; Wadel, P. and Da, P. (2011): Detection of renal function parameters urea & creatinine. Int. J. Pharmaceut. Biol. Arch., 2(2): 734-739.

54. Sherman, K. E. (1991): Alanine aminotransferase in clinical practice. A review. Arch. Int. Med., 151: 260–265.

55. Singh, K. (2013): Evaluation and interpretation of biomarkers of liver diseases. Int. J. Res. Health Sci., 1(3): 213-223.

56. Tahan, G.; Akin, H.; Aydogan, F.; Ramadan, S. S.; Yapicier, O.; Tarcin, O.; Uzun, H.; Tahan, V. and Zengin, K. (2010): Melatonin ameliorates liver fibrosis induced by bile-duct ligation in rats. Can. J. Surg., 53(5): 313-318.

57. Tenhunen, R.; Marver, H. S. and Schmid, R. (1969): Microsomal heme oxygenase. Characterization of the enzyme. J. Biol. Chem., 244(23): 6388-6394.

58. Thapa, B. R. and Walia, A. (2007): Liver function tests and their interpretation. Indian J. Pediatr., 74: 663-671.

59. Udristioiu, A.; Iliescu, R.G.; Cojocaru, M. and Joanta, A. (2014): Alkaline phosphatase isoenzymes and leukocyte alkaline phosphatase score in patients with acute and chronic disease: a brief review. Brit. J. Med. Med. Res., 4(1): 340-350.

60. Udristioiu, A.; Iliescu, R.G.; Cojocaru, M. and Joanta, A. (2014): Alkaline phosphatase isoenzymes and leukocyte alkaline phosphatase score in patients with acute and chronic disease: a brief review. Brit. J. Med. Med. Res., 4(1): 340-350.

61. Whitfield, J. B. (2001): Gamma-glutamyl transferase. Crit. Rev. Clin. Lab. Sci., 38:3263–3553.

62. Whitfield, J. B. (2001): Gamma-glutamyl transferase. Crit. Rev. Clin. Lab. Sci., 38:3263–3553.

63. Williamson, M. A., Snyder, L. M., & Wallach, J. B. (2011). Wallach's interpretation of diagnostic tests (9th ed.). Philadelphia: Wolters Kluwer/Lippincott Williams & Wilkins.

64. http://sunflowerlab.net/patient_preparation.php

65. http://www.merckmanuals.com/professional/appendixes/normal-laboratory-values/blood-tests-normal-values#v8508814

66. http://www.webmd.com/

67. http://www.dovemed.com/

ABOUT THE AUTHOR

Ayman Saber Mohamed was born in Giza, Egypt, in 1984. He received the B. Sc. degree in chemistry and zoology from faculty of science, Cairo University, Egypt, in 2011. He joined the Faculty of science, Cairo University as a Demonstrator in 2013. In 2014, he got the M. Sc. degree and became teacher assistant of molecular and integrated physiology.

www.ingramcontent.com/pod-product-compliance
Lightning Source LLC
Chambersburg PA
CBHW071818170526
45167CB00003B/1354